I0775271

DETOX DIET FOR SENIORS

The Ultimate Detox Guide for
Your Golden Years
Transformation into a Sugar
Free Journey, Energy Boost,
Blood Purification and a Healthy
Liver

Shirlene roberson

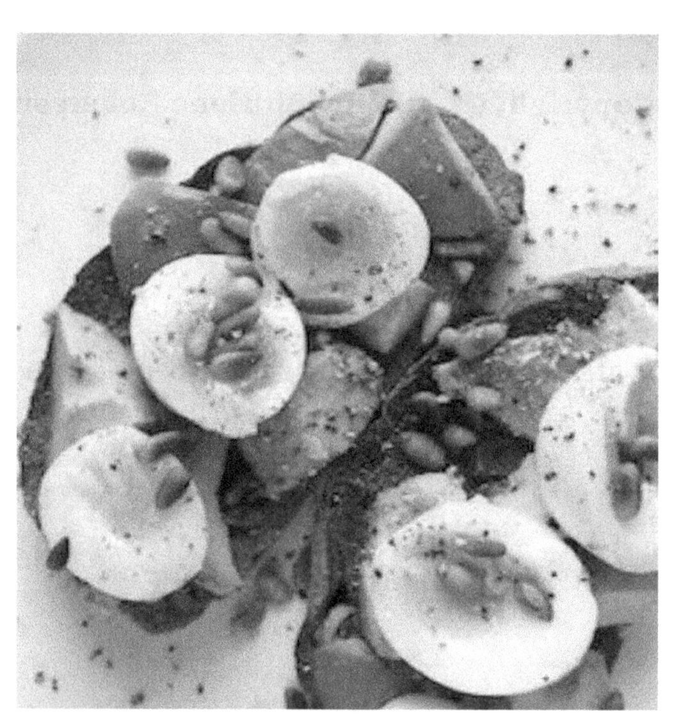

TABLE OF CONTENT

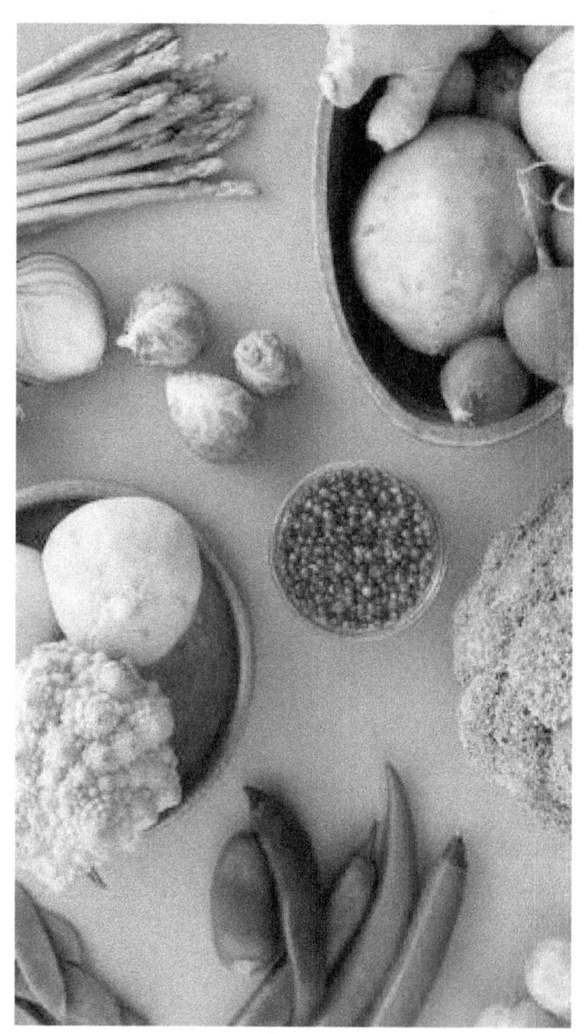

INTRODUCTION

Welcome to Your Health Transformation

Your senior years should be a chapter of vitality, well-being, and profound satisfaction in the golden fabric of life. Greetings and welcome to "**Detox Diet for Seniors**," a thorough manual created to be your reliable travel companion while you restore your health and embrace the energy that accompanies aging.

It becomes more and more clear how important it is to take care of our bodies as we negotiate the complex paths of aging. This book is not only about diets; it's about a revolution in health, a whole-person approach that explores the complexities of how our bodies work and flourish.

Recognizing the Senior Detox Advantages

It is imperative that we understand the significant advantages that detoxification may provide in the context of our senior years before we set out on this life-changing adventure together.

Permit me to share this couple's incredible tale. William and Evelyn Turner was a delightful elderly couple who resided in the sleepy village of Harmonyville once upon a time. Together, the two had spent decades enjoying life's sweetness, laughing together, and conquering obstacles. As their golden years came to an end, they discovered that they were longing for a fresh feeling of health and vigor.

William and Evelyn found an interesting item in the local newspaper one leisurely Sunday afternoon while enjoying herbal tea on their veranda. "The Amazing Power of a Senior Detox Diet" was the headline. The pair was intrigued and looked more, learning that there was a chance for better digestion, increased energy, and general well-being.

Encouraged by the idea of living a better lifestyle, William and Evelyn made the decision to go on a detox trip that would not only improve their physical health but also raise their emotional and spiritual states.

Equipped with shopping lists full of colorful fruits, leafy greens, and healthful grains, the couple emptied their cabinet of processed foods and sweet treat items. As they excitedly experimented with new recipes, experimenting with healthy ingredients that promised to cleanse and revive, the scent of fresh produce filled their kitchen.

Weeks passed, and William and Evelyn saw a slow change in themselves. Their joint aches subsided, their afternoon naps turned into times of quiet contemplation, and their walks in the mornings became more energizing. As the couple relished each mouthful of their revitalizing meals, the previously routine chore of meal preparation became a shared venture, strengthening their bond.

William and Evelyn's faces were glowing brightly, and friends and relatives noticed. Neighbors in Harmonyville were intrigued by the couple's makeover and started asking questions about the key to their renewed energy. Motivated, the Turners made the decision to share their experience by arranging potluck dinners and community seminars to teach others about the life-changing potential of a senior detox diet.

It's never too late to start a path toward wellness and fresh vigor because William and Evelyn's shared experience not only helped them revive their own lives but also sparked a health movement that touched the hearts of a whole town.

We will examine the empirical evidence and practical benefits that a well-designed detox program can provide you. This book is a road map to realizing the full potential of your health, from boosting important organs like the liver to improving mental clarity and energy levels. It's a call to rediscover your vitality and recapture the happiness and energy that should characterize your golden years.

Come along as we explore the realm of senior-friendly detoxification, where every chapter serves as a springboard to a more energetic, healthier version of you.

Are you ready to make a change in your health? Now let's get started.

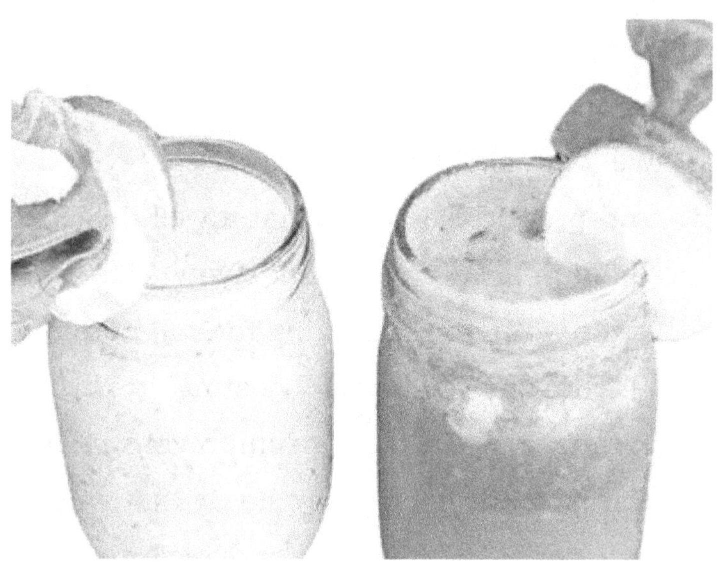

CHAPTER 1

The Detox Advantage for Seniors: A Winning Strategy for Wellness

Starting your golden years is a special chapter in life, and this Chapter lays everything out by explaining why detoxification is not only advantageous but essential at this time. In this chapter, we'll dig into the many benefits of detoxification for seniors as well as the skill of customizing detox for the best possible health in later life.

Investigating the Significance of Detox in the Golden Years

- ***Environmental Toxin Accumulation:*** Seniors may have been exposed to a variety of environmental toxins over time. These may build up in the body and be a factor in health issues. Detoxification becomes an essential method for getting rid of these poisons that have built up, promoting general health.

- ***Reducing Oxidative Stress:*** Chronic illnesses and hastened aging may be caused by oxidative stress, which seniors are often more prone to. With its emphasis on lowering inflammation and eliminating free radicals, detoxification emerges as a potent ally in the fight against oxidative stress.

- ***Supporting Organ Function:*** As we age, our bodies' ability to function as detoxifying organs—like the liver and kidneys—may be compromised. Senior detoxification programs make sure these organs get the support they need to perform at their best and maintain the body's internal equilibrium.

- ***Increasing Energy Levels:*** The amount of energy in seniors may vary. By assisting in the elimination of toxins that cause lethargy, detoxification helps to maintain vigor and energy well into old age.

- ***Mental Clarity and Cognitive Health:*** Detoxification and cognitive health are related. A detox program that supports mental clarity may be beneficial for seniors, perhaps lowering their risk of cognitive decline and improving their general state of brain health.

- ***Encouraging Bone and Joint Health:*** Bone and joint health may be impacted by aging. Removing inflammatory compounds from the body promotes joint health, which enhances mobility and comfort in day-to-day activities.

- ***Mild Approaches to Detox:*** Compared to younger people, seniors may need a more mild approach to detox. Choosing techniques for the detox plan that are both efficient and mindful of the body's innate cycles and possible sensitivities is essential.

- ***Hydration Emphasis:*** Elderly people often worry about being dehydrated. Senior detox plans include drinking enough water to help the body's natural detoxification processes and to improve kidney function.

- ***Nutrient-Dense and Easy-to-Digest meals:*** Senior detox diets have to focus mostly on meals that are both nutrient-dense and simple to digest. This guarantees that the body gets the nutrients it needs without overtaxing the digestive system.

- ***Including Anti-Inflammatory Foods:*** To enhance joint health and lower inflammation and promote general comfort and well-being, senior-specific detox regimens may include an emphasis on anti-inflammatory foods.

- ***Mindful Movement and Exercise:*** Mindful movement and mild exercise are included into senior tailored detox programs. This improves the body's natural detoxification processes by promoting lymphatic fluid circulation in addition to supporting physical wellness.

- ***A Holistic Approach to Mental Health:*** Senior health greatly depends on mental health. Senior detox programs include techniques that support emotional equilibrium, mental clarity, and stress reduction.

It becomes clear that detoxification is not a one-size-fits-all idea as we examine the detox benefit for seniors in this chapter. By customizing detox for the special requirements and benefits of older citizens, we open the door to a health path that celebrates old age, boosts energy, and guarantees a full and active life.

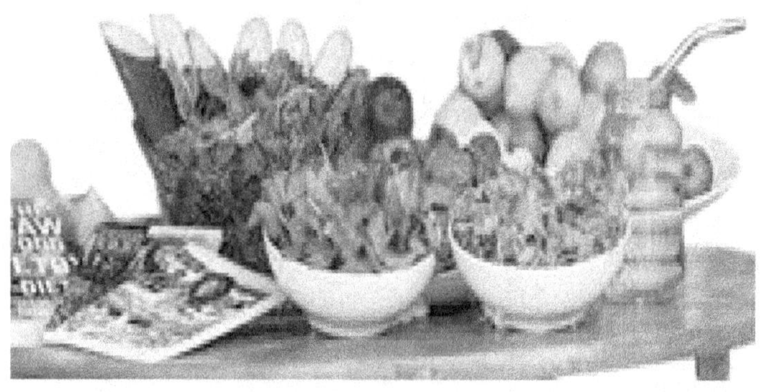

CHAPTER 2

Detoxification Fundamentals: A Path to Wellbeing

Though it's often misunderstood, detoxification is a necessary process that your body goes through on its own. This chapter will demystify the detoxification process, revealing its complexities and exploring how it serves as the foundation for a dynamic and health-conscious way of living.

Detoxification: A Comprehensive Overview of the Body's Harmony

Detoxification is a beautifully arranged symphony played by your body's organs, not a passing fad or esoteric practice. The key players are broken down as follows:

➢ ***The Liver (the Conductor)***: The liver plays the lead role in the detox orchestra. Toxins are converted into molecules that are soluble in water by it, making them ready for excretion. This detox master makes sure dangerous toxins are eliminated before they have a chance to cause trouble.

➢ ***The Kidneys (The Filtration System):*** Consider the kidneys as very thorough filters. Urine is formed as they filter the blood, removing waste and surplus fluid. This ongoing filtering process is a subtle but essential detoxifying procedure.

➢ ***The lungs (the breath of fresh air):*** By allowing oxygen to enter the body, they power cellular functions and facilitate the removal of pollutants. As a result of this complex dance, carbon dioxide is released during exhalation, which aids in the removal of waste.

> ***The Intestines-(eliminators):*** Waste passes via the intestines, where meals high in fiber are essential. Fiber is a key component of the body's detoxification process because it binds to toxins and helps the body eliminate them via stools.

> ***The Skin (The Pores of Release)****:* Heat or physical exertion cause sweating, which allows the skin to release toxins. Our biggest organ, the skin, is vital to the detoxification process yet is often overlooked.

It is false to believe that detoxification is a one-size-fits-all process when you comprehend this symphony. Rather, it emphasizes the body's natural capacity to continually cleanse itself with the correct circumstances and assistance.

How Detoxification Helps Maintain a Healthy Lifestyle: Vitality Building Blocks

Detoxification is a continuous process that is entwined with general health rather than an isolated occurrence. Let's examine how this detoxification process works in tandem with a healthy, balanced lifestyle:

> ➢ ***Enhanced Vitality and Energy:*** When pollutants are removed, energy channels open up. This renewal results in higher energy levels, which promote a bright and vivacious attitude.
> ➢ ***Better Digestive Health:*** A successful detox depends on a healthy digestive system. Adopting a diet high in fiber promotes regular

bowel movements, which help to remove waste and prevent toxic compounds from building up.

> ***Mental Focus and Clarity:*** Cognitive function may be impacted by toxins. By lowering the cognitive burden brought on by accumulated waste, detoxification fosters mental clarity and improves attention and cognitive function.

> ***Beautiful Skin and Age-Wellness:*** The state of the skin is an indicator of the inside. You can promote healthy aging and a bright complexion by assisting detox processes. One of the main causes of early aging is oxidative stress, which is lessened by the method.

> ***Metabolic balance and weight control:*** clearing the body of toxins promotes healthy metabolic functions, which helps with weight

control. Detoxification creates a basis for sustaining a healthy weight by maximizing organ function.

> ***Immune System Resilience:*** The immune system is strengthened by a clean interior environment. By ensuring that the body is prepared to fight against outside dangers, detoxification promotes resilience and lowers the risk of disease.

> ***Harmonious Feelings and Stress Mitigation:*** There is no denying the link between the mind and body. Rejuvenated tissues are more capable of managing stress, fostering resilience and emotional equilibrium.

Essentially, detoxification is a way of living that aligns with the body's natural abilities rather than a band-aid solution. It is an ongoing, dynamic process that establishes the foundation for long-term well-being when given assistance.

Imagine detoxification—rather than a complicated program, as we explore the levels of detoxification in this chapter—as a celebration of your body's innate intelligence, a symphony of energy that beats in time with a healthy way of life.

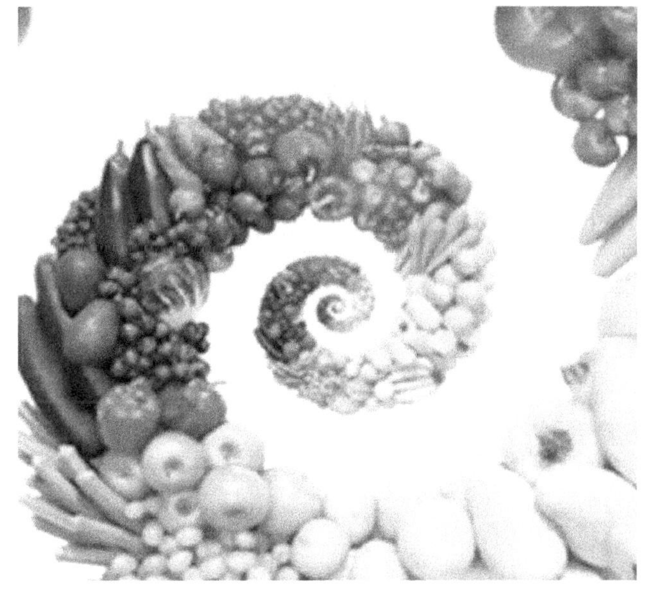

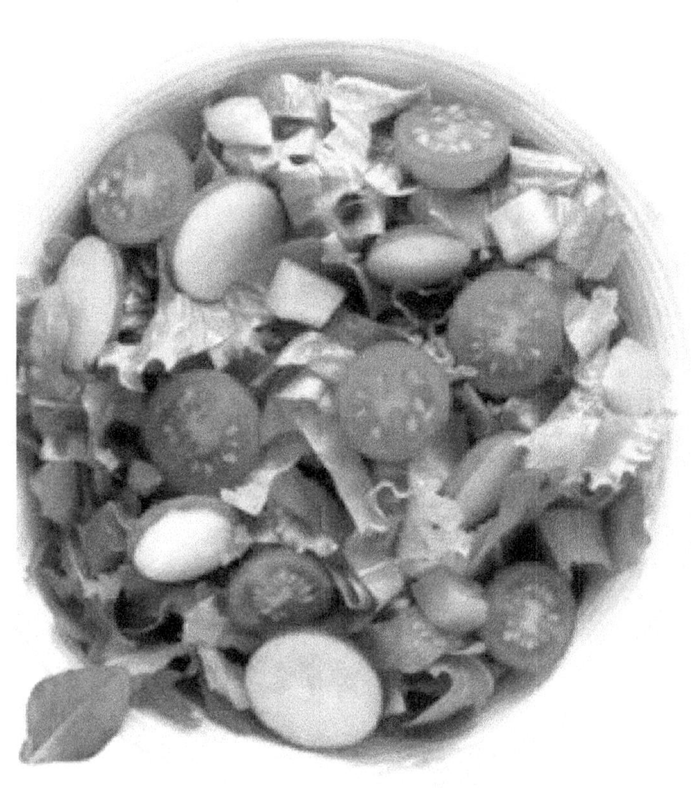

CHAPTER 3

Evaluating Your Health Needs and Customizing Detox for Your Well-Being

When it comes to using detoxification to achieve a healthy lifestyle, the one-size-fits-all method often fails. Personalized detox is complicated, and Chapter 3 is a compass that helps you navigate it by highlighting how important it is to take your unique health circumstances into account. We explore the need of seeking advice from medical specialists in order to guarantee a secure and efficient path to wellbeing.

When detoxification is customized, it becomes an experience made specifically to meet your own health requirements. Here is a thorough examination of important variables to take into account:

- **_Medical Background and Current Health Issues:_** Examine your medical history first. Allergies, chronic illnesses, and drug usage may all have a big impact on the detoxification process. Instead than aggravating pre-existing health concerns, modify your approach to accommodate and assist them.
- **_Understanding your nutritional requirements:_** while accounting for food choices, intolerances, and inadequacies is important.

Formulating a detox regimen high in vital nutrients guarantees the best possible nutrition throughout the purging phase.

- ***Lifestyle and Activity Levels:*** Take into account your everyday pursuits and fitness regimens. A customized detox fits in perfectly with your routine, giving you the energy you need to keep up with your responsibilities each day and maximizing the health advantages of exercise.

- ***Stress Intensities and Mental Health:*** Acknowledge how stress affects your general health. It is crucial to customize your detox to include methods for managing stress and activities that promote mental well-being. Being mindful, unwinding, and getting enough sleep become essential elements.

- ***Status of Hydration:*** Detoxification begins with proper hydration. Evaluate your current level of hydration and modify your detox plan to suit your body's unique requirements for water consumption. Sufficient hydration facilitates the removal of pollutants via several channels.

- ***Detox Objectives and Length:*** Clearly state your objectives for the detox, including weight loss, heightened vitality, or targeted health enhancements. Set a reasonable schedule for your detoxification process and make sure it fits your goals and way of life.

<u>*Seeking Advice from Medical Experts for a Safe Detox*</u>

The cooperation of healthcare providers is essential to a safe and successful detoxification process. This is why their knowledge is so valuable:

- ***Comprehensive Health Assessment:*** Medical practitioners carry out comprehensive health evaluations, accounting for your past medical history, present state of health, and individual health objectives. This thorough assessment guarantees that the detox program is tailored to your specific requirements.
- ***Medication Review and Adjustments:*** If you use medication, medical specialists may examine your prescription and make

necessary adjustments to the detox plan. By doing this, possible interactions are avoided and it is made sure that the detox process enhances rather than replaces current therapies.

- ***Monitoring Vital Signs:*** Blood pressure, heart rate, and metabolic indicators may all be tracked with routine check-ins with medical specialists. This continuous evaluation guarantees that the detoxification procedure stays secure and does not jeopardize your general well-being.

- ***Advice on Nutritional Requirements:*** Medical experts provide advice on how to satisfy your nutritional requirements while going through detox. This contains suggestions for supplements to support the body's processes and avoid deficiencies, if needed.

- ***Handling Detox negative Effects:*** There may be short-term negative effects from detoxification. Healthcare providers can support you through this, including techniques for coping with pain and making sure that any negative responses are dealt with right away.

- ***Developing a Sustainable strategy:*** Working with medical experts allows for the development of a detox strategy that goes beyond the first stage. By limiting the recurrence of pollutants, they may help build durable lifestyle modifications that enhance long-term well-being.

Personalized detox is essentially a collaboration between your medical team and yourself. Through consultation with experts and alignment with your specific health requirements, you set out on a safe and customized road to maximize your well-being. It is essential to highlighting how crucial it is to comprehend your health situation and get professional advice in order to have a cleanse that really speaks to your unique personality.

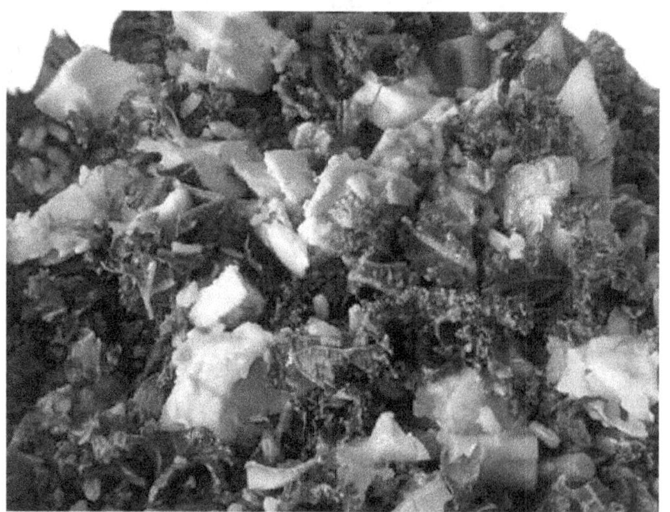

CHAPTER 4

Developing Your Detox Strategy: Personalized Wellbeing for Seniors

In this Chapter, we'll be focusing on creating a detox program specifically for seniors. This chapter explains how to create a detox diet that is suitable for seniors and emphasizes the need of include nutrient-rich meals for the best possible outcomes. Together, we will set off on a health path tailored to the unique requirements and energy of the elderly.

> ***Recognizing the Nutritional Needs of Seniors:***

Lean Proteins: To maintain and rebuild their muscles, seniors need a sufficient amount of protein. Lean items like fish, chicken, tofu, and lentils are your best bet.

Calcium and vitamin D: are necessary for healthy bones. Get your calcium from dairy products or fortified foods, and get your vitamin D from supplements or sunshine.

Foods High in Fiber: Fiber from fruits, vegetables, and whole grains supports digestive health by promoting regular bowel movements.

<u>***Good Fats:***</u> For heart health, give priority to unsaturated fats from nuts, seeds, avocados, and olive oil.

> ➢ ***Making Hydration a Priority:*** The feeling of thirst may diminish with age, which raises the risk of dehydration. Incorporate hydrating meals like melons, cucumbers, and soups into the detox regimen and emphasize the use of water.

> ➢ ***Considerate Calorie Consumption:*** The calorie requirements of seniors may vary. Create a detox plan that will help you stay within a healthy weight range and yet have enough energy for everyday tasks.

> ➢ ***Embracing Anti-Inflammatory Foods:*** To promote joint health and general well-being, include foods with anti-inflammatory qualities,

such as berries, turmeric, ginger, and leafy greens.

> ***Reducing Processed Food and Sodium Intake:*** Seniors often worry about heart health and lowering their risk of hypertension, so cut down on processed foods and sodium.

Including Nutrient-Rich Foods for the Best Outcomes

Berries for Antioxidant Power: High in antioxidants, blueberries, strawberries, and raspberries help to maintain cognitive function by preventing oxidative stress.

Omega-3 Fatty Acids from Fatty Fish: To get omega-3 fatty acids, which are good for the heart and brain function, eat fatty fish like salmon or trout.

Leafy Greens for Vital Nutrients: Swiss chard, kale, and spinach are rich in vitamins and minerals that are important for strong bones, a healthy immune system, and vitality.

Cruciferous Vegetables for Detox Support: The liver's detoxification activities are supported by certain substances found in broccoli, cauliflower, and Brussels sprouts.

Whole Grains for Sustained Energy: For critical nutrients and long-lasting energy, choose whole grains like oats, brown rice, and quinoa.

Probiotics for Gut Health: Include fermented foods, yoghurt, and kefir to assist digestion and nutrient absorption by fostering a healthy gut microbiota.

Herbal Teas to Help with Hydration and Detoxification: Select teas with hydrating qualities and possible detoxifying effects, such as chamomile, ginger, or dandelion.

Nutrient-Dense Snack alternatives: Nutrient-dense and filling snack alternatives include almonds, walnuts, and fresh fruit slices.

Seniors may start a detox program that works for them by carefully choosing and mixing these nutrient-dense meals. This chapter provides guidance by exposing the range of tastes and nutrients that go into creating a detox diet that is suitable for older adults. In order to ensure that seniors succeed in their health journey, a strategy that not only supports the body's natural detoxification processes but also improves overall vitality is being developed.

CHAPTER 5

Seniors' Sugar Detox: Recognizing Sugar's Effect on Elderly Health

It's important for seniors to know how sugar affects their health as they start their path toward better health. Sugar intake has been connected to a number of health problems, and elderly people may be more susceptible to its negative effects. Here are some key considerations:

> ➢ ***Control of Weight:*** It might be difficult for seniors to maintain a healthy weight. Consuming too much sugar increases the risk of weight gain and obesity, which may worsen pre-existing medical conditions.

> ***Health of the Heart:*** Consuming a lot of sugar is linked to a higher risk of heart disease. Seniors should be aware of their cardiovascular health, and cutting less on sugar may help lower cholesterol and blood pressure.

> ***Risk of Diabetes:*** Type 2 diabetes is more likely to occur in older adults. Consuming too much sugar may aggravate insulin resistance, which is a risk factor for diabetes. Controlling sugar consumption is crucial for both managing and preventing diabetes.

> ***Mental Process:*** Sugar has been connected to a higher risk of dementia in older people as well as cognitive deterioration. A low-sugar diet may lower the risk of neurodegenerative illnesses and improve cognitive performance.

➢ **Bone Well-Being:** Consuming a lot of sugar may harm bone density and cause diseases like osteoporosis. Seniors must maintain optimal bone health in order to avoid fractures and preserve their mobility.

Realistic Techniques for Cutting Sugar Consumption

- **Examine food labels:** Seniors should learn how to read food labels well in order to spot hidden sugars. If ingredients like sucrose, high-fructose corn syrup, and other sweets aren't carefully examined, they can slip missed.
- **Opt for Whole Foods:** Generally speaking, whole, unprocessed foods have less added sugar. Seniors should concentrate on include

nutritious grains, lean meats, and
fresh produce in their diet.

- ***Minimize Drinks with
  Sweeteners:*** A large portion of the
  daily sugar consumption comes
  from sugary beverages. To keep
  hydrated, seniors can choose sugar-
  free beverages like water or herbal
  teas.

- ***Select Natural Sugar Substitutes:***
  In moderation, seniors may choose
  natural sweeteners such as honey,
  maple syrup, or stevia as needed.
  These choices provide sweetness
  with less detrimental effects on
  health.

- ***Gradual Inversion:*** Seniors may
  cut down on sugar gradually as
  opposed to trying a sudden sugar
  detox. This strategy makes changing
  one's lifestyle more sustainable.

- ***Maintain Hydration:*** Maintaining enough hydrated helps reduce cravings for sugary foods. Seniors should make it a goal to stay hydrated throughout the day.
- ***See a Nutritionist for Advice:*** Seniors who want to reduce their sugar intake might benefit from working with a nutritionist to create a realistic and customized strategy. This guarantees that dietary modifications correspond to personal health requirements.

In conclusion seniors are better able to make decisions when they are told about the effects of sugar on their health and are given doable methods for cutting down on their consumption. Seniors may start a sugar detox that supports general well-being and lifespan by taking a deliberate and progressive approach.

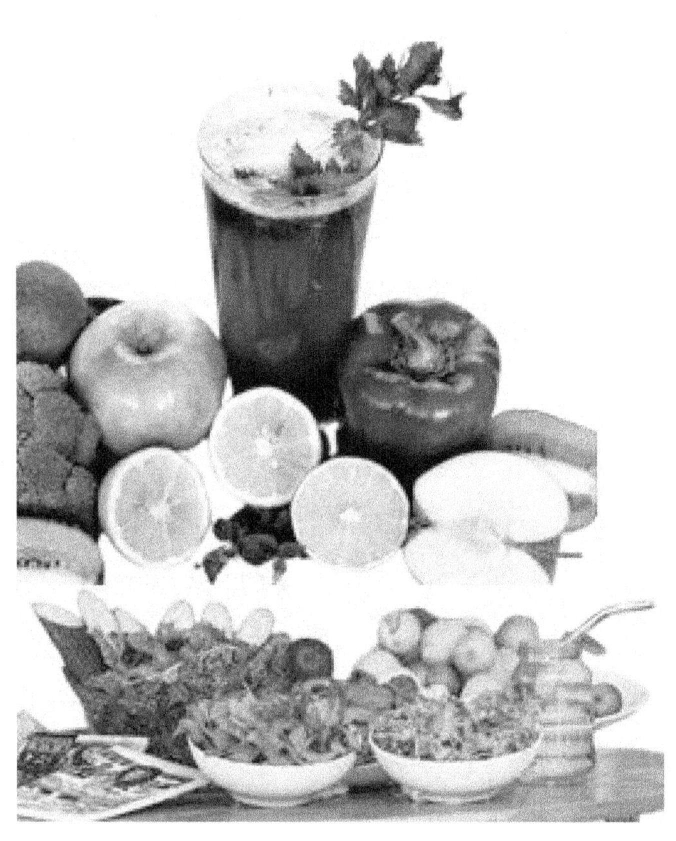

CHAPTER 6:

Seniors' Detox: Nourishing the Liver

The Liver's Crucial Function in Detoxification - one essential organ that is essential to the body's detoxification process is the liver. Comprehending the functioning of the liver is crucial for seniors who prioritize their health and start a detoxification process.

> ➢ ***Procedure for Detoxification:*** Toxins, medications, and other dangerous compounds that enter the body are processed and neutralized by the liver. Maintaining general health depends on this detoxification process, particularly as the body ages.

> ***Nutrient Storage and Metabolism:*** Seniors' diet-related nutrition metabolism is handled by the liver. It maintains a constant supply of vital vitamins and minerals for the body's operations.

> ***Control of Blood Sugar:*** Blood sugar management may provide a barrier for elderly individuals. In order to balance blood sugar and avoid dangerous surges, the liver helps control glucose levels.

> ***Metabolism of Fat:*** The liver is essential for the production of energy and the breakdown of lipids. Elderly people need to support the function of their livers since poor fat metabolism may lead to a number of health problems.

> ***Foods Rich in Nutrients:*** A diet high in fruits, vegetables, whole grains, and lean meats should be the first priority for seniors. Antioxidants and vital minerals included in these meals promote liver function as well as general health.

> ***Drink plenty of water:*** Adequate hydration is crucial for the health of the liver. To support the liver's activities and aid in the removal of toxins, seniors should strive to consume a sufficient quantity of water each day.

> ***Teas made with herbs:*** Some herbal teas, such milk thistle and dandelion root tea, are well-known for supporting the liver. These teas

are tasty and healthy drinks that seniors may enjoy on a regular basis.

➢ ***Eat Less Processed Food:*** Preservatives and chemicals found in highly processed meals might put stress on the liver. Seniors should consume less processed meals and instead prioritize complete, natural foods.

➢ ***Moderate Intake of Alcohol:*** Drinking too much alcohol might be especially bad for the liver. Depending on their health, seniors should strive for moderation or think about cutting out alcohol from their diet.

➢ ***Consistent Exercise:*** Exercise promotes general health, which includes liver function. Seniors may improve their liver health and blood circulation by doing little exercise, swimming, or strolling.

➢ **_Steer Clear of Overeating:_** Heavy, large meals may strain the liver. To aid in digestion and lessen the strain on the liver, seniors can concentrate on portion management and space out their meals throughout the day.

➢ **_Frequent Medical Exams:_** Regular health examinations are essential for assessing liver function. Seniors and medical professionals should collaborate closely to identify and quickly treat any possible liver problems.

Nourishing the liver is a fundamental aspect of a senior's detox journey. By understanding the liver's vital role in detoxification and adopting habits that support its health, seniors can enhance overall well-being and contribute to a successful and sustainable detoxification process.

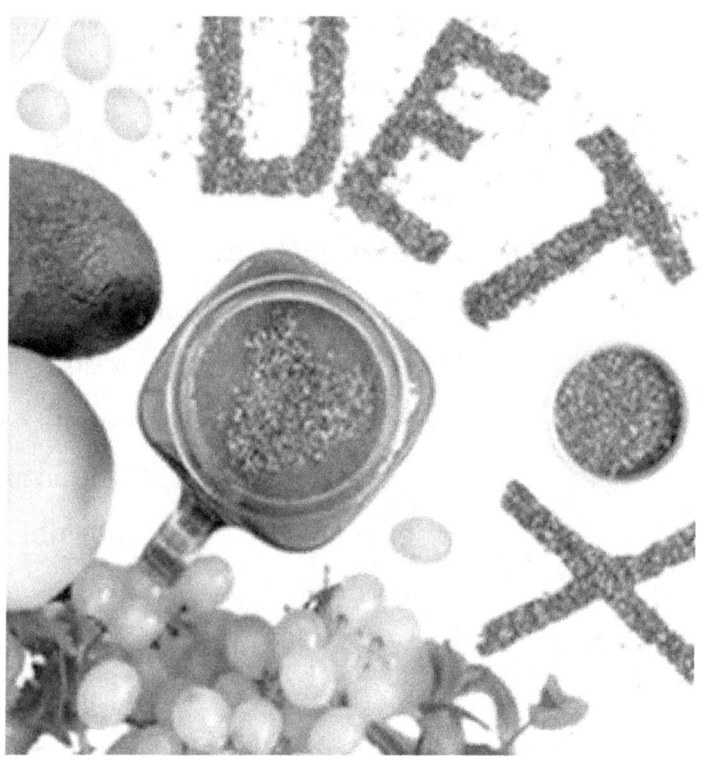

CHAPTER 7

Blood Balance for Improved Health

To balance blood health, controlling seniors' Blood Sugar Levels is vital by:

- ***Being Aware of Blood Sugar:*** Blood sugar management is a common problem for seniors. High blood sugar levels have been linked to a number of health conditions, such as diabetes and heart difficulties.

- ***Blood Sugar Control Is Important:*** For seniors, controlling blood sugar levels is critical to avoiding problems including weariness, cognitive impairment, and an elevated risk of infections. It is especially important during a detoxification process since normal blood sugar levels promote general wellness.

- ***Diet High in Nutrients:*** A diet rich in nutrients that includes whole meals that release glucose gradually is the main emphasis for seniors. In order to assist regulate blood sugar levels, this includes diets high in fiber, lean proteins, and complex carbs.

- ***Consistent Meal Schedule:*** Setting regular mealtimes may assist in controlling blood sugar levels. To minimize fluctuations and crashes, seniors should strive for regular times between meals and steer clear of extended fasts.

- ***Tracking Your Consumption of Carbs:*** Seniors should be aware of the kinds and quantities of carbohydrates they eat, even though they are a necessary source of energy. Choosing fruits, vegetables, and whole grains over processed carbs will help you keep your blood sugar levels stable.

- **Control of Portion:** Blood sugar control requires careful portion control. Seniors may prevent overeating, which can cause blood sugar swings, by using smaller plates and being mindful of portion sizes.

- **Frequent Exercise:** Blood sugar control is significantly influenced by exercise. To increase insulin sensitivity and regulate blood sugar levels, seniors should exercise on a regular basis. Examples of this kind of exercise include walking, swimming, and light weightlifting.

- **Strategies for Reducing Stress:** Blood sugar levels might be impacted by prolonged stress. Seniors may improve their mental health and blood sugar regulation by engaging in stress-relieving hobbies, deep breathing techniques, or meditation.

The Relationship Between Blood Health and Detox

- **Effect of Detoxification on Blood:** Detox programs with a thoughtful design may improve blood health. Detoxification maintains the liver and other organs involved in blood health by focusing on nutrient-dense diets and avoiding processed and sugary foods.
- **Cutting Down on Foods That Inflame:** One common goal of detox diets is to lower inflammation. Foods that cause inflammation

should be avoided by seniors since they may aggravate issues including insulin resistance and poor blood sugar regulation.

- ***Blood circulation and hydration:*** Maintaining enough hydrated promotes blood circulation and is essential to detoxification. Hydrated cells work better, removing waste and facilitating the transportation of nutrients, all of which improve blood health.

- ***Removal of Toxins:*** The liver and kidneys are two organ systems that participate in detoxification processes that help remove toxins from the circulation. This may contribute to lessening the circulatory system's total workload.

- ***Tailored Detox Programs:*** Elderly people should collaborate with medical specialists to create personalized detox regimens that take into account their unique medical requirements and any drug interactions. This guarantees a secure and efficient method for promoting blood health via cleansing.

Part of a thorough senior detox treatment includes balancing blood for optimum health. Seniors may improve general well-being by controlling blood sugar levels via nutrition, frequent exercise, and stress management. The link between blood health and detox highlights the need of a comprehensive strategy that takes into account lifestyle and dietary aspects in order to maintain a healthy circulatory system.

CHAPTER 8

Senior-Friendly Detox Recipes

these delectable and nutrient-dense smoothies, lunches, and snacks are designed to help seniors who are detoxing. Seniors may fuel their bodies and improve overall well-being by consuming a range of nutritious foods high in vitamins, minerals, fiber, and antioxidants. With their variety of tastes and textures, these dishes make detoxing pleasurable and long-lasting. Before making major dietary changes, always get advice from a healthcare provider or nutritionist, particularly if you have a medical condition or are on medications.

<u>*Stir-fried quinoa with vegetables:*</u>

Ingredients

- Cooked quinoa
- a variety of vibrant veggies (carrots, broccoli, and bell peppers)
- lean protein (shrimp, tofu, or chicken)
- For flavor, add ginger and garlic.
- Tamari or low-sodium soy sauce

Directions:

- Stir-fry protein and veggies in a skillet with ginger and garlic.
- Include the cooked quinoa and mix to thoroughly incorporate.

Packed with fiber, protein, and antioxidants, this dish helps seniors maintain their detoxification process while giving them vital nutrients.

Sweet Potato Roasted with Baked Salmon:

Ingredients

- Wild-caught salmon fillets
- sweet potatoes, peeled and diced
- lemon juice, olive oil, and herbs (thyme, rosemary); salt and pepper for flavor

Directions:

- Marinate salmon with herbs, lemon juice, and olive oil.
- Bake fish and serve it over roasted sweet potatoes, providing antioxidants and omega-3 fatty acids.

- Roast sweet potatoes with a splash of olive oil, salt, and pepper.

Vegetable Lentil Soup

Ingredients

- Rinsed and dried lentils
- Various veggies (carrots, celery, onions)
- Vegetable broth with low sodium content
- Seasoning with coriander, cumin, and garlic

Directions:

- Simmer veggies and lentils in vegetable broth.
- Garlic, cumin, and coriander are used to season.

- This fiber-rich soup supports digestive health and provides essential nutrients for a satisfying meal.

Stuffed Peppers with Quinoa and Turkey:

Ingredients

- Lean ground turkey
- Quinoa
- Green bell pepper
- Tomato sauce and Italian herbs

Directions

- Cooked turkey and quinoa mixing with tomato sauce and herbs.
- Bell peppers should be stuffed and baked till soft.

- This meal is rich in protein, provides a well-balanced combination of tastes and nutrients.

Chickpea and Vegetable Salad

Ingredients

- Mixed greens
- Roasted chickpeas
- grilled veggies (zucchini, eggplant, cherry tomatoes)
- Feta cheese and balsamic vinaigrette

Directions

- Mix together roasted chickpeas, grilled veggies, and mixed greens.
- Top with feta crumbles and balsamic vinaigrette drizzle.

- This light salad offers plenty of vitamins and minerals, fiber, and protein.

Five Smoothies and Snacks to Strengthen Your Detox Process

Kale or spinach for the Green Detox Smoothie:

- Celery, cucumber, and green apple
- Water or coconut water
- Ginger and lemon juice

Directions*: Blend all ingredients until smooth. Rich in hydrating qualities and antioxidants, this green smoothie aids in the body's detoxifying processes.*

Greek Yogurt Parfait

- Greek yogurt

- Berries (strawberries, blueberries)
- granola and honey drizzl

Directions: *Top with Greek yogurt, berries, and granola. Drizzle with honey to create a tasty and nourishing parfait.*

Humus dip and avocado

- Ripe avocado
- Hummus
- Whole-grain crackers or vegetable sticks

Directions*: Mash avocado and combine with hummus; serve as a dip for vegetables or whole-grain crackers.*

Chia Seed Pudding

- Chia seeds
- Coconut or almond milk

- A little bit of maple syrup combined with vanilla essence

directions: *Blend chia seeds with milk, maple syrup, and vanilla essence. Chill until pudding-like consistency.*

Roasted Chickpeas

- Rinsed and drained canned chickpeas
- olive oil, spices (paprika, cumin, and garlic powder)

directions: *Roast till crispy to make a filling, high-protein snack.*

Successful Detox-Friendly Meal Planning Advice:

- ➢ *Use Fresh Ingredients:* To optimize nutritional intake and taste, use fresh, whole foods.

- ➢ *Mindful Cooking Methods:* To retain nutrients, use cooking techniques like steaming, baking, or sautéing with little to no oil.

- ➢ *Experiment with Herbs and Spices:* Try enhancing taste with herbs and spices instead of adding more salt.

- ➢ *Remain Hydrated:* To aid with detoxifying, include foods high in water content, such as fruits and vegetables, into your meals.

- ➢ *Customize Recipes:* For a more individualized approach to detox-friendly meals, modify recipes to suit specific tastes and nutritional requirements.

CHAPTER 9

Developing Exercise Mastery to Enhance Your Detox Experience

Exercise's transforming potential becomes apparent as a dynamic force throughout the thrilling detoxification trip, helping you move toward a refreshed and revitalized version of yourself. This chapter walks you through the fine art of striking the ideal balance as it reveals the complex tango between physical activity and older citizens. Get ready to be astounded as we explore workout methods that have been carefully designed to enhance the cleansing process.

<u>*Elderly People and Exercise: Finding the Harmonious Balance*</u>

Our seniors enter the physical exercise stage to the sound of a symphony of movement. The secret is to find a rhythm that synchronizes with your body's specific requirements, not to push limits. Imagine a soft dance that combines power and suppleness, with choreography that honors the knowledge that has been accumulated over time while also igniting energy.

Break free from the illusion that physical ability declines with aging. Accept customized programs that honor years of experience, combining strength training, flexibility drills, and low-impact aerobics into a unique motion symphony. See how the body effortlessly yields to the call of movement, bringing latent energy to life and guiding poisons toward a quick departure.

Workout Methods for Detoxification: Exposing the Craftsmanship

> ➢ **_Yoga Alchemy:_** Dive into the age-old practice of yoga, which is a carefully crafted symphony of poses and breathing techniques. Asanas that massage internal organs and stimulate detoxification pathways include the cleaning twists and energizing inversions. Feel the energy flowing, letting go of the weight that has built up within.

> ➢ **_Cardiovascular Euphoria:_** Boost your heart rate and cleanse your body by engaging in cardiovascular exercises that make your heart race. Imagine walking briskly, cycling, or doing water aerobics and feeling the

surge of endorphins washing away pollutants from your system. With every beat, the body, now a canvas of ecstasy purges.

➢ **The Renaissance of Resistance Training:** Seniors, revel in the wonders of personalized resistance training. Your creative tools will be resistance bands and light weights, which will help you sculpt strength and remove toxins from your body. This deliberate opposition creates a vibrant, resilient work of art.

➢ **Mindful Tai Chi Movement:** Take a trip through elegant motions with Tai Chi, a martial art turned captivating dance. The methodical, slow movements strengthen muscles, improve balance, and cultivate an awareness of one's body. Toxins make a discrete departure as you move elegantly through the shapes.

In this chapter, we rethink exercise as a beautiful painting where purification and ageing meet. Seniors, be ready to fall in love with movement again, with the transforming methods described here acting as paintbrush strokes on your freshly awakened energy. Accept the relationship between age and fitness, overcoming boundaries, and allowing your detoxification process be a masterpiece of your creation.

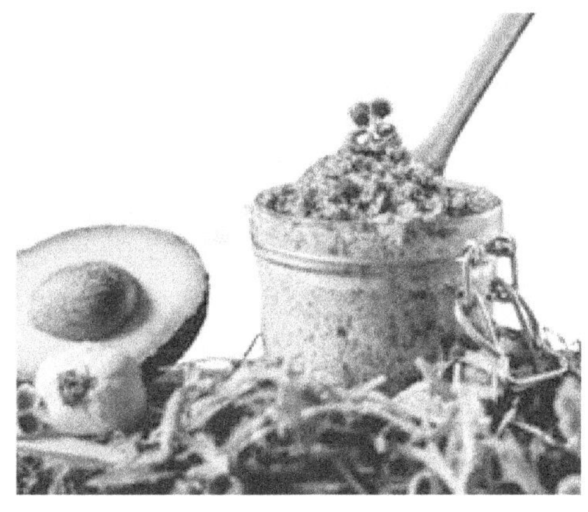

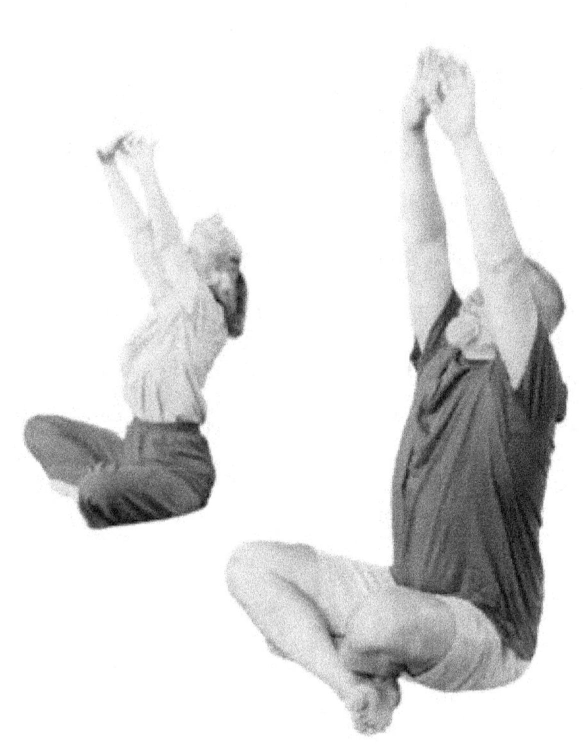

CHAPTER 10:

Mindful Liberation: Revealing the Potential of Emotional and Mental Detoxification

Detoxification on the mental and emotional levels plays a crucial role as the mastermind behind holistic health in the larger scheme of things. By dissecting the mind-body relationship, this chapter reveals the significant influence of emotional wellness on geriatric health. Get ready for an adventure into the worlds of stress relief and mindfulness, where techniques open out like flowers and each one has its own special scent of peace.

Imagine the mind as the captain of a vessel sailing the currents of life, while the body as the vessel itself. The symbiotic relationship between physical and mental health intensifies in later life. Seniors, take note of this: emotional health is the ship's compass, not just a passenger.

> ➢ ***Neuroplastic Symphony:*** Accept the idea of neuroplasticity, in which the brain's capacity for self-rewiring emerges as a ray of hope. Take part in mental activities that increase cognitive function and build mental toughness and dexterity. The instruments of this symphony include puzzles, memory games, and picking up new abilities;

together, they create a song of renewal.

> ***Awareness as the Guide:*** Enter the calm of mindfulness, a discipline that turns the present moment into a haven. Seniors: practice awareness by taking thoughtful walks, deep breathing exercises, and meditation. A peaceful sea of clarity replaces mental clutter as you ground your consciousness in the present moment.

Techniques for Reducing Stress and Improving Emotional Health: Creating Your Own Haven

> ***Emotional Alchemy via Art:*** Harness the healing potential of creative expression. Whether it's writing, painting, or any other creative endeavor, it becomes a way

to let go of emotions. Transform your worries into poetry and your tension into colorful brushstrokes, and then observe as your emotional canvas becomes a work of art.

➢ **Laughing Yoga:** The Happy Rebellion: Fill your days with the ageless joy of contagious laughter. Laughter yoga is a technique that combines breathing exercises with yoga poses and may be used as a means of emotional cleansing. Your being is filled with joyful vibrations that release stress and invite emotional purification.

➢ **Connective Threads of Social Interaction:** Use social ties to weave an emotional support network. Talk to people, join groups, or take part in neighborhood events. The cure to isolation is human interaction, which promotes emotional fortitude and a feeling of community.

> ***Nature's Embrace:*** Give yourself up to the healing power of the natural world. Seniors: take walks in parks, enjoy the sound of falling leaves, and let the wind's soft touch ease your tension. Every stride one takes in nature's haven restores emotional well-being; it is a panacea for the spirit.

Mental and emotional detoxification is more than just an idea in this life-changing chapter; it's a call to find your inner resilience. Let the mind-body connection be a harmonic symphony that resonates with the tempo of your path towards holistic health, seniors. Unlock the secrets of emotional well-being.

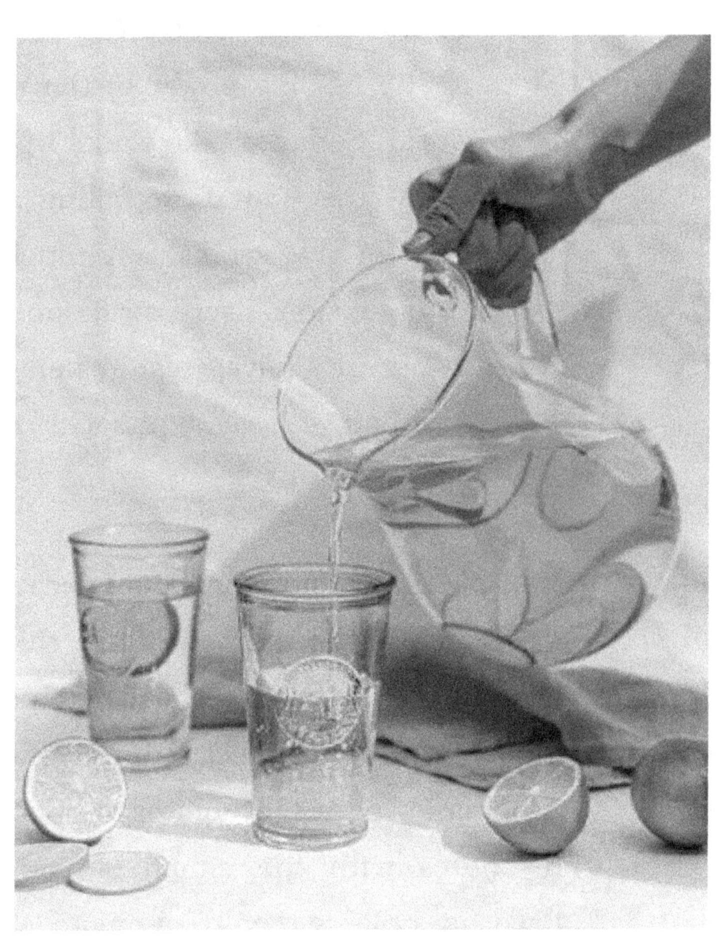

CHAPTER 11

Overcoming Adversities: Handling and Overcoming Detox Obstacles

Starting a detoxification journey is a brave step toward health, but it's not always easy. Chapter 11 outlines the typical obstacles that may occur and offers a strategy for getting beyond them. Get ready to strengthen your determination as we explore the nuances of taking on obstacles head-on and maintaining motivation throughout the detox journey.

Typical Obstacles and Solutions: Mapping the Terrain of Detox

- **Physical Discomforts:** Headaches, exhaustion, or changes in digestion may be brought on by detoxification. Do not be alarmed; they are often fleeting indications of the body adjusting. To ensure a safe and successful transition, stay hydrated, do light workouts, and think about speaking with a healthcare provider.

- ***Cravings and Withdrawals:*** Say goodbye to the comforting pull of go-to delights as cravings and withdrawals try to take over. To overcome this obstacle, use strategic planning. To satisfy cravings, provide nutrient-dense substitutes, and consult a nutritionist to create a meal that is both filling and suitable for a detox.

- ***Social Temptations:*** Social events and festivities, often focused on decadent meals and libations, weave the fabric of society. Equip yourself with boldness and tenacity, and let friends and family know what your detoxification objectives are. Seek companionship from others who share your dedication to health.

- ***Time Restraints:*** Adopting a detox program may be difficult given the hectic nature of contemporary living. Don't be afraid; time may be your devoted buddy. Make time for exercise, plan your meals in advance, and include mindfulness into your everyday routine. Over time, perseverance turns into the triumphant song in this dance.

Maintaining Your Motivation During Your Detox Process: Creating an Inner Fire

- ***Goal Visualization:*** Construct a clear, detailed mental image of your final objective. Imagine the refreshed you, experiencing more vitality, mental acuity, and general well-being. This graphic road map serves as a motivating compass, assisting you in navigating obstacles and diversions.

- ***Honor Milestones:*** Divide the trip into more manageable, joyous benchmarks. Every day, every week, and every accomplishment is worthy of recognition. Celebrate your accomplishments and allow them to inspire you to take on the next difficulties.

- ***Empower and Educate:*** Information is a powerful friend. Learn about the science of detoxification and its enormous effects on health. By expanding your comprehension, you provide yourself with the knowledge necessary to make wise decisions, providing a strong basis for your commitment.

- ***Mindful Reflection:*** Take regular breaks to consider how your path has changed. Pay attention to the changes that are occurring in your body and mind. Your commitment to the detox road is reinforced by the little changes—whether they be mental, emotional, or physical—which act as quiet confirmations of your progress.

This chapter tackles the shadows that come with the detox trip and turns them into resilience-building stepping stones. Obstacles turn into chances for development, and drive becomes the steadfast light illuminating the way to overall well-being. Seniors, use this chapter as a roadmap to help you overcome obstacles and come out on top of your detoxification journey.

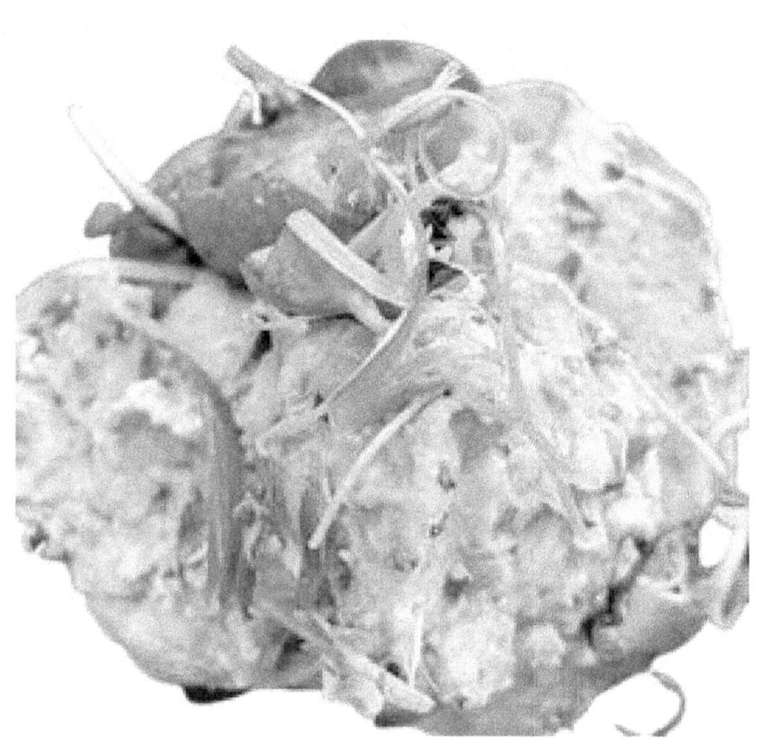

CONCLUSION

The culmination and continuation of detoxification victories

It's time to recognize our accomplishments and map out a plan for long-term wellbeing that goes beyond detox as this life-changing adventure draws to an end. This last chapter delves into the significant importance of acknowledging your detoxification accomplishments and assisting you in making the shift to an eternally healthy lifestyle.

Honoring Your Detox Achievements:

Highlighting the Wins

- ***Reflecting on the Journey:*** Give
  yourself a minute to consider the
  amazing journey you have just
  completed. Think back to the
  difficulties encountered, the
  fortitude shown, and the changes
  seen. This reflection is an
  acknowledgement of your strength,
  dedication, and the importance of
  self-care—it's more than simply a
  retrospective.

- ***Gratitude and Self-Appreciation:***
  Develop an attitude of appreciation
  for your body's flexibility and
  resiliency. Recognize the beneficial
  changes that have occurred on the
  inside as well as the outside and
  appreciate the devotion put into the
  detox process. Give yourself plenty
  of gratitude for your path, which
  demonstrates your dedication to
  living a better, more fulfilling life.

- ***Celebration Rituals:*** Commemorate your detox's conclusion with heartfelt customs. Create memories that celebrate the trip and mark the start of a new chapter in your life, whether it's a peaceful stroll in the outdoors, a healthy spa day, or a straightforward get-together with loved ones.

Maintaining Your Health After the Detox: Maintaining Your Glow

- ***Applying Lessons to Everyday Life:*** The knowledge acquired throughout the detoxification process is a gold mine for enduring wellbeing. Incorporate the workout regimens, mindfulness exercises, and dietary advice into your everyday life in a seamless manner.

Allow them to serve as the cornerstone of your lifelong quest for wellness.

- ***Changing Dietary patterns:*** Even if the detox may have made you eat in a cleaner, more conscious manner, keep changing your eating patterns. Adopt a varied, nutrient-dense diet and enjoy the tastes of healthful foods that support long-term energy and nourishing your body.

- ***Fitness as a Lifestyle:*** The workouts that drove your detoxification process are not just regimens; they are routes to lifelong health and wellbeing. Integrate fitness into every aspect of your life by trying new things, appreciating diversity, and cultivating an enduring love of movement.

- ***Mindfulness as a Daily Practice:***
  You don't have to wait till the detox
  phase to experience the peace that
  comes with mindfulness. Make
  mindfulness a way of life rather
  than just a technique. Take regular
  breaks for focused breathing,
  deliberate presence, and silence to
  ground yourself in the peace that
  you have developed during your
  detox.

- ***Creating Holistic objectives:*** After
  the detox, create objectives that are
  comprehensive and address mental,
  emotional, and physical health.
  Whether your objectives are to learn
  a new skill, develop stronger
  relationships, or follow a passion, let
  them serve as a compass to help
  you live a happy and meaningful
  life.

Let the joy of finishing this purification journey serve as a springboard for a future full of energy and wellbeing, rather than merely serving as a symbol of accomplishment. Seniors, as you close this chapter on your trip, keep in mind that health is a lifestyle that is a continuous and thriving journey rather than a destination. May the light of your health always shine on the pages that are yet to be written.

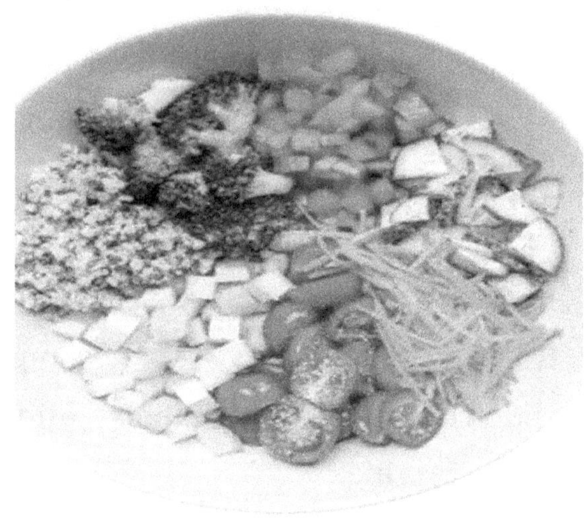

BONUS

10 Simple And Easy To Prepare Natural Drinks And Juices For Detoxification.

1. Lemon water: squeeze the juice of half a lemon into a glass of warm water. This simple drink helps to cleanse the digestive system and promote hydration.

2. Green tea: brew a cup of green tea and let it cool. Green tea is rich in antioxidants and can aid in detoxification by supporting liver function.

3. Cucumber and mint infused water: slice a cucumber and add it to a pitcher of water along with a handful of fresh mint leaves. Let it infuse overnight in the refrigerator.

This refreshing drink helps to flush out toxins and promote hyderation.

4. Beetroot and carrot juice: blend together one beetroot and two carrots with a little water. This juice is packed with antioxidants and can support liver health

5. Ginger and turmeric tea: grate a small piece of ginger and a teaspoon of turmeric into a cup of hot water. Let it sleep for a few minutes before drinking. This warming tea has anti-inflammatory properties and can aid in detoxification.

6. Watermelon and mint smoothie: blend together chunks of watermelon and a handful of fresh mint leaves with a little water or ice. This refreshing smoothie is hydrating and can help flush out toxins.

7. Pineapple and ginger juice: blend together fresh pineapple chunks and a small piece of ginger with a little water. Pineapple contains enzymes that aid digestion, while ginger has anti-inflammatory properties.

8. Cranberry and orange infused water: mix together cranberry juice and freshly squeezed orange juice in a glass of water. Cranberries are known for their detoxifying properties, and oranges provide a boost of vitamin C.

9. Aloe Vera juice: blend the gel from an Aloe Vera leaf with water and a squeeze of lemon juice. Aloe Vera has natural detoxifying properties and can support digestive health.

10. Blueberry and spinach smoothie: blend together blueberries, spinach and a banana

with a little water or almond milk. Blueberries are rich in antioxidants, while spinach provides essential nutrients for detoxification.

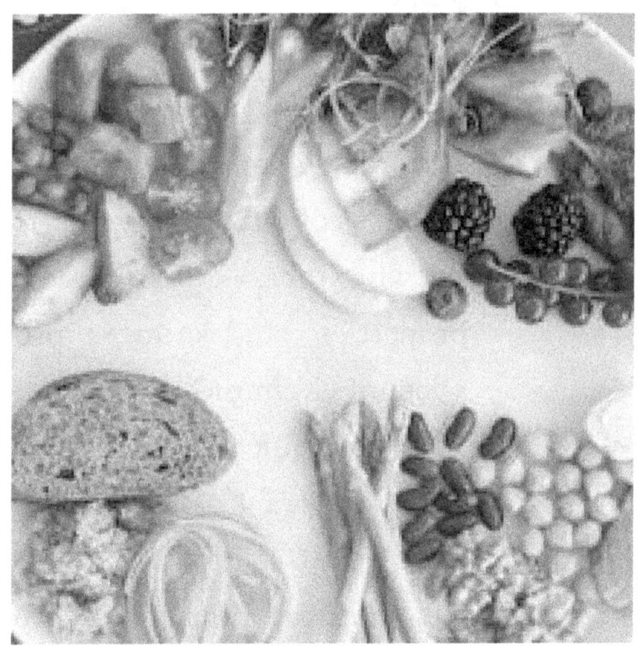

THANK YOU FOR READING.